Turn Medicaid Nightmares into Miracles

Turn Medicaid Nightmares into Miracles

Let's Deal with Medicaid and Protect Your Assets - NOW!

Cheryl L. Fletcher-Docherty

With Steve Marsh

To order additional copies of this book, contact:
Xlibris Corporation
1-888-795-4274
www.Xlibris.com
Orders@Xlibris.com
108326

DISCLAIMER:

We consider it essential that readers of this book obtain professional legal, accounting, tax and Medicaid planning advice before attempting to implement concepts presented in this book; laws vary state by state and according to federal law in all matters covered in this book and need such guidance to assure proper understanding within Medicaid guidelines. This book was written to provide the most insightful and accurate information possible regarding Medicaid planning and related issues, but all information contained within is subject to changes, revisions and new legislation pertaining to Medicaid rules and regulations. Information about Medicaid policies and procedures in this book may become outdated or rendered incorrect by official rulings. Laws and rules currently regarding the nature of trusts, real estate, real estate law, annuities and other items mentioned in this book may change at any time, thus rendering the information in this book inaccurate. No individual annuity products or annuity carriers are recommended, promoted or favored over others in this book; examples of the use of so-called Medicaid-appropriate annuities are included in a hypothetical context only; before purchasing any annuity, professional financial Medicaid-related advisory, legal and tax consultation must be sought to assure applicability within ever-changing state and federal guidelines. The author(s) and publisher assume no liability whatsoever from individuals acting upon the advice disseminated in this book; the aforementioned professional advice must be used to assure the most effective use of concepts suggested in this book as potential strategic models for Medicaid planning. No guarantees are offered by the author(s) or publisher that individual Medicaid employees would accept or approve applications based on advice and insights offered in this book; decisions made by Medicaid employees may be arbitrary and unpredictable in nature, and therefore cannot be predicted or guaranteed.

Before you begin to read my book, let's dispel some Medicaid mythology:

Some people think that most Medicaid beneficiaries are on Welfare.

This is anything but true! In fact:

- Anyone with US citizenship can receive Medicaid. You do not have to be poor.

- People I have helped to acquire Medicaid benefits were not on welfare; they would not have needed me if they were on welfare.

- The vast majority of Medicaid beneficiaries have assets to protect before joining the Medicaid program.

- Medicaid beneficiaries who have gone into the system through me are on Medicaid because I have repositioned and protected their assets.

READ THIS BOOK AND YOU WILL NOT BE IMPOVERISHED BY MEDICAID.

CONTENTS

FOREWORD

By Bill Kanter

J.D., M.B.A.

TRUE STORY (Of course the names have been changed): Lois came to see me a few days after she admitted her husband Sam into a local nursing home. She was quite emotional. Both in their early 70's, Lois and Sam had raised two beautiful daughters, paid off their home and had saved over $600,000 for their retirement. They lived modestly, invested conservatively (they did not lose money in the stock market in 2001-2003 or in 2008) and were looking forward to spending their golden years together.

At age 71 Sam was diagnosed with dementia and quickly lost the abilty to function on his own. Lois could not take care of him at home—they did not have long term care insurance which could have paid for care in their home—so she took him to the nursing home. Lois toured the nursing home and liked the place and then sat down with the administrator who told her, and her daughters, that the cost at that home was **$9,000 per month!!** No, that is not a misprint!

It did not take Lois more than a few seconds to realize that in a little over five years their nest egg money would be gone. Then she would have to sell their house—worth about $300,000—and after three more years of nursing home payments she would be left with absolutely nothing, at which point Sam could qualify for Medicaid so the government would pay nursing home expenses for him. This is why Lois was emotional.

Fortunately for Lois, a family friend and retired attorney whom I know told her to seek the advice of a Medicaid planning attorney and she called me. After listening to about 15 minutes of her story I told her not to worry because she would pay the first month's payment of $9,000 to the nursing home and then **she would not have to pay them anymore**. I told her that we could get Sam qualified for Medicaid.

Lois did not believe me at first but that is exactly what happened. **Now, years later, the Government is still paying for Sam's care and Lois has kept all of her money.**

If you have a family member or loved one that is in a nursing home or needs to be in one and you want to get Medicaid to pay for them, then navigating the complex and arcane universe of Medicaid is extraordinarily difficult. The Supreme Court has acknowledged that the Medicaid statute is "an aggravated assault on the English language, resistant to attempts to understand it." (Schweiker v. Gray Panthers, 453 U.S. 34,43 (1981). However if you are reading this book you should feel blessed.

Cheryl L. Fletcher-Docherty is God's gift to you. You might think this is over the top praise but then again, you have not seen the tears of joy shed, and the blessings said, once the Lois's of the world speak to her. When Cheryl told me she was writing a book in plain English, to help the average person qualify for Medicaid, I was thrilled.

I have seen Cheryl spend an entire day at the convention of the National Academy of Elder Law Attorneys (NAELA) educating Elder Law attorneys who do not know much about Medicaid qualification law. More important for you, the people who read this book, I have heard her speak to the Lois's of the world and reassure them that there is always a way to protect some, or often all, of their assets. Cheryl's knowledge of the Medicaid rules and benefits—and how to access or apply for them—far exceeds any other Medicaid planner or attorney in the country. Her caring and ability to explain complex laws in a down to earth manner is exceptional.

I have read Cheryl's book and I consider it an extremely valuable resource for anyone navigating the Medicaid application process. As she says (exhaustively) throughout the book, it is essential to have qualified legal assistance when actually implementing any of these strategies.

Lois recently came by my office so I could help her fill out the simple annual Medicaid redermination form. She also gave me a gift and she told me how much better her life is, now that she does not have to worry about giving all of her money to the nursing home. She still goes to see Sam every day, she is just much less emotional about it.

This is just one example of how quality Medicaid planning can improve the lives of people across the nation.

Bill Kanter, J.D., M.B.A.
Member: National Academy of Elder Law Attorneys (NAELA)
www.illinoismedicaidattorney.com

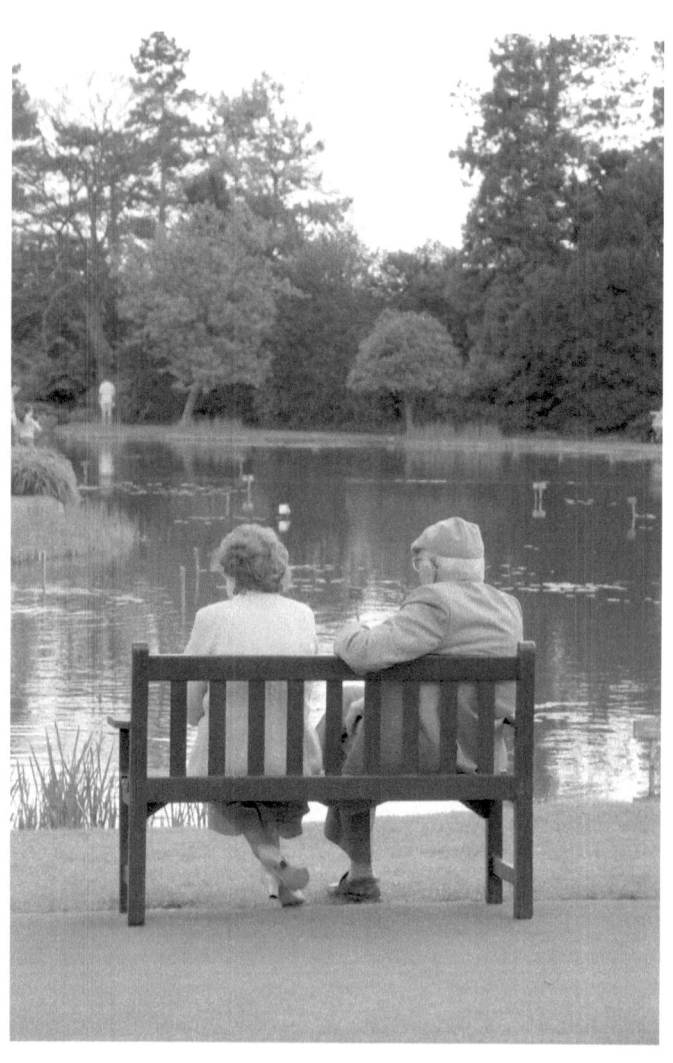

INTRODUCTION

Welcome to Strategic Medicaid Planning!

By Cheryl L. Fletcher-Docherty
Medicaid Planning Specialist

I F YOU HAVE not yet faced the infuriating, mind-boggling, Byzantine nightmare awaiting most Americans embarking upon the Medicaid qualification system, you probably will—unless you have so much money that unnecessarily losing a fortune will have little effect on your life.

For the rest of us, the certainty we face no matter how much money we have—or don't have—is that Medicaid qualification almost *never* happens overnight without proper planning.

Without proper, strategic planning for Medicaid qualification, the sad reality is that already cash-strapped families will face enormous hospital and nursing home bills on behalf of loved ones in need, and they will likely lose everything in the process.

Middle-income and wealthy families will similarly stand by, watching in helpless dismay as entire estates and inheritance legacies vanish before their eyes.

As for the wealthy, I have never met a well-to-do family that wanted to leave a significant portion of its estate to hospitals, nursing homes or the state, especially when they found that such losses could be avoided! Yet, vast fortunes are being lost every day through poor Medicaid planning. Even more tragic are hard-working American families forced into bankruptcy due to the lack of advance Medicaid planning.

Let's face it: Most of us have no "vast" fortune to fall back on when a medical crisis strikes a loved one. As a result of poor planning, the real tragedy accordingly occurs when *entire* family legacies are stripped away—sometimes within a few short months or even weeks—because an elderly loved one falls into "the zone" of nursing homes and exploding hospital costs for catastrophic care.

Such legacies—meaning inheritance money earmarked for a grandchild's education, or retirement legacies meant for adult children of the stricken elderly—have all too often been quickly consumed by bloated and quickly rising nursing home costs, hospital expenses and other sources of virtually unlimited potential for *complete* financial annihilation.

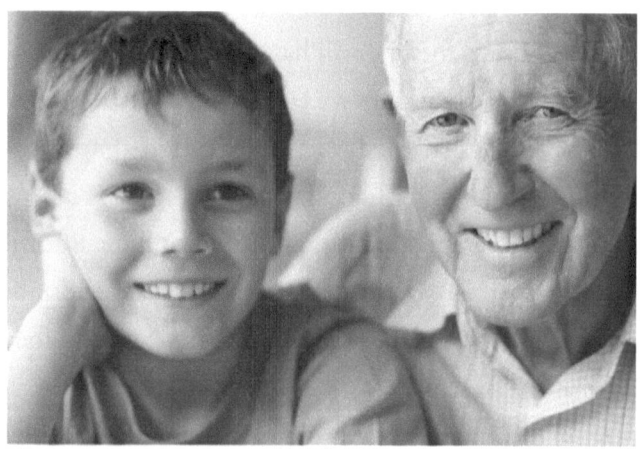

Statistically, this kind of annihilation happens DURING the Medicaid application process itself—the often lengthy period that occurs *before* benefits are ultimately approved. This happens because, without solid Medicaid planning, a stunning mountain of fees will overwhelm family savings virtually overnight. Why?

Let's look at a hypothetical client based on case files in my office. Here I present Pam, an elderly widow, and her adult children Sean and Megan.

Pam falls in the bathroom of her own home one night and breaks her hip. Never mind that she lies in agony over an entire weekend and nearly dies of dehydration—the bathroom sink standing above her like an unapproachable monolith. No, the real saga begins after Pam is safely in the hospital recuperating and accumulating ever-mounting hospital expenses. Never mind the fact that no one will inform Sean and his sister Megan about the brief, 100-day period during which Pam will be covered by Medicare—*and that Pam will be held responsible for a large Medicare co-pay.*

While some of the co-pay costs will be paid by Pam's health insurance policy, coverage limitations leave Pam with a disturbing portion of other out-of-pocket expenses.

Yet, the real nightmare begins immediately after the 100-day period of Medicare coverage comes to an end—after it is obvious that Pam will need long-term care in a nursing home.

Without warning and according to procedure, when Medicare coverage runs out, the hospital packs Pam into an ambulance and sends her to a nursing home for continued care. At the same time, Megan and her brother Sean assume that Medicaid coverage will automatically kick in at the nursing home, simply because they started the Medicaid application process while Mom was still in the hospital.

Never assume anything during the Medicaid application process!

First, no one bothered to check the status of the nursing home itself. Does the home accept Medicaid patients? Not this one, unfortunately, so Pam will have to be moved after Sean and Megan spend a grinding week in search of a nearby nursing home willing to accept Medicaid patients. Meanwhile, Pam is racking up an astounding bill for absolutely 100% out-of-pocket nursing home and related medical fees. The Medicaid nightmare has begun in earnest.

Next, unfortunately—and all too typically—Medicaid caseworkers will soon arbitrarily reject Pam's application due to a long list of speed bumps based on little known rules and regulations. Such infractions can easily occur because rules and regulations vary widely from state to state and even county to county. Such "infractions" can even be determined according to the whims of certain Medicaid case workers and the way they view an individual application!

That said, after the fog finally lifts less than two months after Pam initially entered the nursing home, Sean and Megan are horrified by the realities of huge bills from both the nursing home AND the hospital. The nursing home has been merrily charging the national-average monthly fee of $6,500 for Pam's care. Yet, in the middle of her first month in the nursing home, Pam was returned to the hospital for a two-day stay and tests. Her insurance company covered much of the $27,000 hospital bill for the tests, but Pam now faces an additional $4,700 for her part of the insurance co-pay.

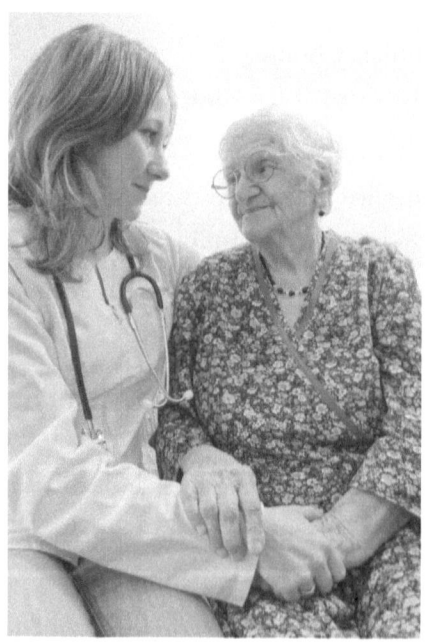

In short, within two months of falling in the bathroom, Pam suddenly owes more than $11,000 to the combined health care facilities, and their ever-efficient bill collection procedures begin almost immediately. Calls from hospital and nursing home collectors make life at home a living hell for Megan, who seems to receive an inordinate share of this legal version of telephone harassment, which creates more than one argument with her brother Sean. In fact, both Megan and her family, and Sean and his new bride, are already squaring off for a feud that will take years to heal. All because Mom assumed that Medicaid would step in and magically "take care of everything."

And the bills keep growing, month after month, as repeated Medicaid applications are repeatedly rejected. By the end of Pam's first 12 months of nursing home care, she owes more than $100,000 out of pocket, which must come from the dwindling $200,000 inheritance that Sean and Megan had hoped to share one day.

By the middle of the following year, nearly the entire $200,000 inheritance will be gone, with the exception of the nominal sum of $2,000 allowed by Medicaid to remain in her bank account. Only then will Pam become eligible for Medicaid.

By then, however, and most ironically, Pam's hip is finally beginning to heal. Another statistical stunner is that a remarkable percentage of Medicaid people—nearly 25 percent—will eventually be declared healed by the nursing home! Like Pam, they will be sent home impoverished. Unlike Pam, many will have homes to return to, but for poor Pam the situation will descend into yet another nightmare. The family will be forced to sell her home to provide her with living expenses, so she will be forced to move in with one of them—a most unwelcome situation all the way around. But it never had to happen this way.

As a highly qualified Medicaid Planning Specialist of more than 15 years, I have run into this type of tragedy time and again. Yet, I have never lost the passion to prevent it, given enough time for advance planning, or to stop the Medicaid destruction cycle in mid-stream.

I'm not sure of the exact date, but I decided to tackle this challenging business after helping a family member and a couple of friends through the process. After enduring the living hell of traversing a Medicaid jungle of cubicles and offices, red tape and often conflicting rules and regulations, a number of patterns and behind-scenes procedures became clear to me. I began to see how the whole mish-mash of Medicaid rules and procedures actually fit together—not just locally, here in southern California, but nationwide as well.

From my seaside office in Santa Cruz, I now field questions from people all over the nation in need of solving their individual Medicaid nightmares. These people include average folk who become my clients and they include elder law attorneys, estate lawyers and financial planners from every corner of the U.S.—all of whom run into seemingly incomprehensible hurdles in the Medicaid application process.

After all these years, I can tell you one thing: Advance Medicaid planning WILL make all the difference. I can also say that even after the axe falls due to a lack of advance planning, there ARE Medicaid planning tactics and strategies that can be applied to stop the hemorrhaging of money being lost to health care providers and nursing homes.

In this book, I cover both advance and after-the-fall Medicaid planning strategies that you will be able to use RIGHT NOW—to either prevent the nightmare or stop it in its financially lethal process.

If you read this book in its entirety, I guarantee that you will know far more than you do now about the facts—and the financially crippling myths—surrounding Medicaid.

For a great number of Americans who are either impoverished, in the hard working middle class, or among the wealthy segment of our nation, Medicaid will one day become your reality. So let's get started right now.

CHERYL L. FLETCHER-DOCHERTY

If you are in the middle of the nightmare, take a deep breath and start tackling Medicaid with my help and the facts in this book: You need to know that real solutions exist, RIGHT NOW. And if you have the luxury of time to plan, take the information in this book and ACT NOW, before a health care nightmare robs you of every unnecessary cent you will lose through the lack of proper planning.

Now, all you have to do is turn the page and begin the learning process!

Most Sincerely,

Cheryl L. Fletcher-Docherty
Medicaid Planning Specialist

Asset Preservation Strategies
1307 West Cliff Drive
Santa Cruz, CA 95060
Email: Cheryl@MedicaidAnnuityPlanning.com
Web site: www.MedicaidAnnuityPlanning.com

CHAPTER 1

How Medicaid Works—
Things You *Must* Know

Impoverishment Made Easy . . .
Through Lack of Planning

F OR SOME PEOPLE, the following numbers are a real shocker: Looking at the statistical make up of all residents in nursing homes, and other long term care facilities, Medicaid pays up to *only* 45% of total long term care costs, while Medicare pays 14% and standard health insurance policies pay 11%. So, Medicaid is not THE end-all solution for long-term care, but for many it is the only solution available.

Too many people are forced to give everything they own to nursing homes while waiting for Medicaid benefits to kick in. This is one reason why "out-of-pocket" expenses among residents of long-term care facilities make up an astounding 23 % of nursing home revenues. Scary, right?

Let's put a face on the figures based on adult children Sean and Megan, and Megan's mother Pam, who suddenly faces life in a nursing home any day. Pam will be required to pay all of her own nursing home expenses until she qualifies for full Medicaid coverage. At an estimated $6,500 per month—the average monthly nursing home fee in her state—Pam's entire retirement nest egg of $150,000 will go to the nursing home in less than two years. Only then, when she is nearly flat broke, will she "possibly" qualify for Medicaid.

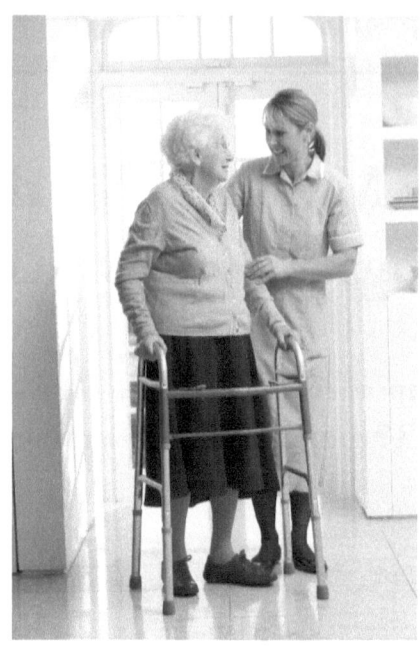

I say she will "possibly" qualify because a number of critical speed bumps could *indefinitely* extend her waiting period for Medicaid acceptance—even though she is flat broke, except for an allowable $2,000 (in most states) in her bank account.

I point to Pam's all-too-common dilemma because there are people out there who will never go on Medicaid, because they never seek proper planning in advance. They will pay out of pocket for the remainder of their lives until they run out of money. This is called "Medicaid spend-down." That's right, you "spend-down" everything you own until you're flat broke, which sounds fine to some people, but what if your health improves and you are declared "well" enough to be discharged from the nursing home. This happens, although the more likely scenario leaves your surviving spouse or a favorite heir with nothing after you die.

Yet, Pam's typical financial crisis can easily be avoided. Had she been savvy enough to initiate a strategically compliant Medicaid plan in the beginning, she would have been able to minimize, or even eliminate, her own out-of-pocket payments to the nursing home and qualify for Medicaid benefits immediately.

The ABCs of Medicaid Spend-down:

Once you've reached what both the state and federal government consider "impoverishment," once you've reached the level of having no more than $2,000 to your name—if you are single, non-married or a widow—only then will Medicaid pick up your medical and long term care costs. People with more than $2,000 are forced to spend the excess—and I mean everything from stocks and bonds to pensions and real estate—until your assets dwindle "down" to $2,000 or less.

What many people tragically fail to understand is that "spend-down" does not always exclude transferred or gifted assets. More often than not, people are shocked to find that gifted assets are countable and must be spent down—or the value of such gifts are added to your Medicaid waiting period before you may qualify for Medicaid benefits. While waiting for the perceived value of your improperly gifted assets to be counted, you continue to pay out of pocket for your nursing home care. Improperly transferring or gifting assets to a son or daughter, or anyone other than your spouse, including transferring a home—or even titling your home—in the name of one's children, is not a permissible transfer in the eyes of Medicaid.

In terms of Pam's home, for example, if she does not transfer her home to Sean and Megan everything will be fine. *Medicaid will allow her to keep her own home* and still receive Medicaid benefits because the home is considered exempt.

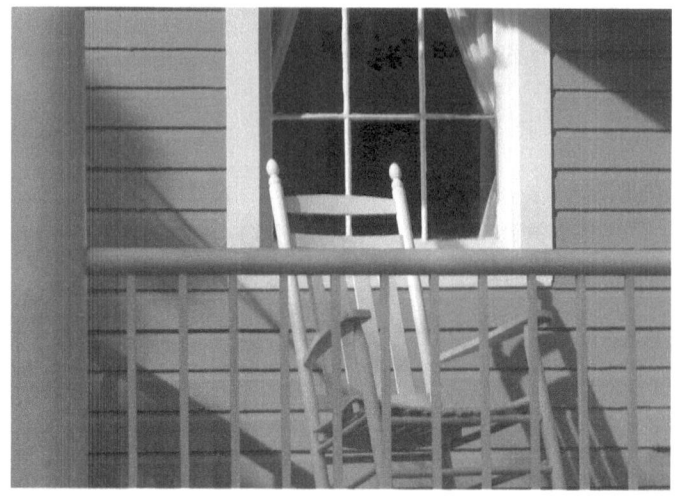

In general and in most states, the house is excluded if the equity value is below $500,000 (the permissible equity value may be greater in some states). However, if she does transfer her home to Sean and Megan, Medicaid declares the home an "uncompensated" transfer if Sean and Megan do not pay Pam what the home is worth, say, $200,000. If Medicaid considers the home an uncompensated transfer, Pam will be penalized for that entire amount.

In other words, Medicaid will add the $200,000 value of the home to the total amount owed for spend-down. Pam will NOT be eligible for Medicaid until she pays that amount, or until she "spends-down" that amount by being denied Medicaid coverage for a certain period of time, which is called a "penalty period" typically equating to several months or years.

Each state has its own equation to determine the penalty period created by improperly transferred assets. The equation—called a Divestment Penalty Divisor (DPD)—is often based on the average cost of nursing home care in that state. If, for example, the average cost of nursing home care is

$6,500 per month, Medicaid coverage would be denied for 30 months according to the state's DPD, due to the transfer of Pam's home to Sean and Megan!

Again, every state is different. In Florida, for example, the state's calculated average cost of nursing home care is only $5,000 per month, which extends her penalty period. The transfer of the $200,000 house would cause Pam to be ineligible for Medicaid for a penalty period of 40 months, if she were a Florida resident.

I can't say it enough: During that 40-month period, Pam would have to self-pay, or privately pay, her own nursing home costs for 40 months before Medicaid would start picking up the tab.

As a qualified Medicaid Planning Specialist I always advise people to avoid this kind of mistake, which is often well-intentioned. One possible consequence of Pam's decision would force Sean and Megan to sell the house in a poor real estate market, or in a strong, buyer-friendly market, where the $200,000 home would sell for only $150,000, which would then be repaid to Pam, who would be forced to use the money for her nursing home costs until she reached impoverishment and, accordingly, qualification for Medicaid coverage. Unfortunately, disastrously, Pam would then be without a home to return to, should she be declared cured and "well" by the nursing home, and ultimately released. In any event, the home would be snapped up by nursing home fees.

Spend-down via Property Rental & Other Options

One option in this scenario—especially in those states that have an unlimited exclusion for income producing property—would be for Pam to rent her home in effort to avoid probate and estate recovery; this may be accomplished by properly structuring the deed so that upon her death it is out of the estate. While rules vary in each state, some—if not most—would consider Pam's home exempt as a rental property. The net rental proceeds would, however, be considered countable as income. The net income is that income received after subtracting all expenses, such as: management fees, assessments, utilities, maintenance, and real estate taxes. As such, you want to make certain that your total income does not equal or exceed the nursing home private pay rate, so that you would still be considered eligible for Medicaid.

Here, it would be especially advantageous to contact a Medicaid Planning Specialist or duly experienced attorney to verify the precise nature of state regulations concerning property rental while receiving Medicaid benefits. Mistakes could lead to penalties, but the rewards of proper Medicaid planning in this area have obvious benefits.

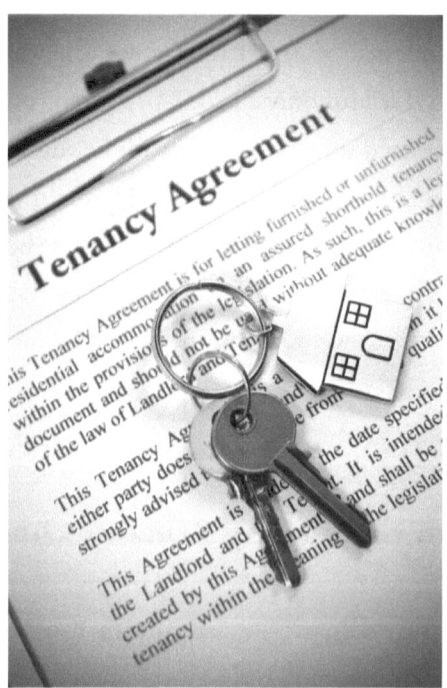

Again, the calculations can be complicated for a novice, but the garnering of rent can be an effective part of Medicaid planning overall.

CHERYL L. FLETCHER-DOCHERTY

Other spend-down options include: paying off/down your existing mortgage; purchasing a home (in 2011 the equity limitation was $500,000 in most states); doing home improvements; purchasing a vehicle, although some states have equity limits; purchasing or upgrading personal property, but be careful not to go overboard with this option; pre-paying funeral and burial expenses, although there are caps on the amount you can use to fund these plans; purchasing a Medicaid compliant annuity, if you are in a state that recognizes this type of annuity in the context of Medicaid planning; purchasing Single Premium "no Cash Value" Life Insurance, if you are in a state that recognizes this type of insurance in the context of Medicaid planning.

Before implementing your own spend-down strategy, always consult an elder law or Medicaid-savvy attorney who would be well familiar with rules within your state. Your Medicaid Planning Specialist may have a directory of such individuals as well.

Your Absolutely Critical "Intent to Return Home"

Another tricky, little-known fact about maintaining the home exemption under Medicaid is to clearly state on the Medicaid application form your "intent to return home" after a stay in the health care system, including the nursing home—no matter how long you believe you may be living in a nursing home or how likely, or unlikely, it may be that you would be able to return home. This is most necessary in order to make sure that your home will remain exempt from Medicaid spend-down. Once you leave your home for the nursing home, it is recommended that you prepare and sign a written statement declaring your intent to return to your home when you are well enough.

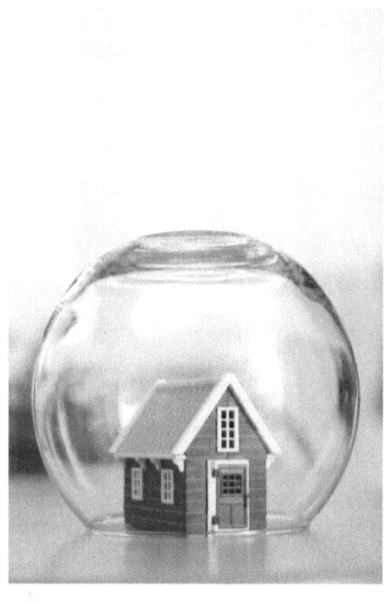

Normally, each state's Medicaid application form will provide a question regarding your intent to return home after your nursing home care. Some states go so far as to provide a separate, official form for you to declare your intent to return home. You would simply check the appropriate box and sign the individual form.

However, some states DO NOT provide such a form or even a place to state your "intent to return home" on the state's Medicaid application. Yet, your statement of intent remains a federal Medicaid regulation. As such, I always like to make certain that the written statement of your intent to return home is included with the Medicaid application.

Without the statement and the continued intent to return home, it would not be unthinkable for some Medicaid administrator to review your case, discover the lack of your statement of intent, and remove your home exemption from Medicaid spend-down, especially after several months or years have passed. This would mean, of course, that Medicaid would stop payment of your nursing home bills until the determined value of your home met the designated Medicaid penalty period.

If you were otherwise impoverished, you would have to quickly sell your home to make your nursing home payments, or you would be asked to leave the nursing home altogether or even involuntarily discharged, a most unpleasant prospect for many patients in need of nursing home care.

Even when states DO provide forms or "intent" sections on application forms, I *still* like to submit an independent statement. In no situation do I give Medicaid case workers the leeway to interpret our intent. This can become a most important safety measure in your ability to maintain ownership of your home *and* future Medicaid coverage.

In short, even if some states fail to provide a place to clearly state your intent to return home after nursing home care, overall federal regulations clearly declare your need to do so, in order to maintain your home exemption. Yes, it's true, and that some states fail to provide a space for declaration is rather unsettling, in my opinion. But that's the way it is, so beware.

Yes, you may never return home. Your medical condition may be such that we KNOW you will never return home. But it doesn't mean that you don't have the "want" or the desire to return home, or the "will" to return home. They cannot take that away from you. So, you owe it to yourself and your survivors or heirs to guard your home exemption.

You must never let a Medicaid case worker say, "Look, we both know the seriousness of your health condition—wouldn't it be true to say you never intend to return home?" Don't be fooled. You must *never* let them talk you out of the home exemption. Be aware that some case workers might just try it, in order to expose your home to spend-down. I've seen case workers verbally question people about their intent, as if to intimidate them into abandonment of the exemption. But again, no matter how sick you are, wouldn't you love to be back at home, rather than in a nursing home?

Who wouldn't jump at the chance to return home due to an unexpectedly positive change of health?

I have had cases, rare cases, where patients with serious illnesses were rehabilitated enough to go home. It happens.

CHERYL L. FLETCHER-DOCHERTY

CHAPTER 2

Medicare *vs.* Medicaid
and
Compliant Assets vs.
Nightmare Annuities

M ANY PEOPLE THINK Medicare will cover them for skilled nursing care if they enter a nursing home, but Medicare covers only Day 1 through Day 20, at full coverage.

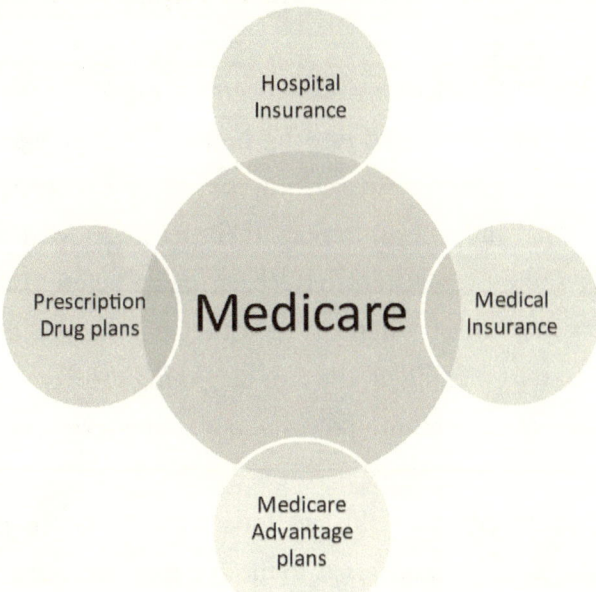

From days 20 through 100, the patient will be required to meet a co-pay under Medicare, and this is even before Medicaid begins. As for the Medicare co-pay from Day 21 through Day 100 in a skilled nursing facility, you would pay $144.50 per day in 2012. If you are in a nursing home charging $200 per day, payment of the additional $58.50 would be your responsibility.

I get a lot of concerned clients who call a bit shocked, saying they thought they would be fully covered for at least 100 days under Medicare, but they find, to their dismay, that they really are not fully covered during the latter 80 days of the Medicare period.

After that, Medicare is completely out of the picture: Beginning on Day 101, you are on your own. You will be 100% responsible for all of your nursing home costs and fees, which will quickly spiral into the thousands and even hundreds of thousands of dollars without Medicaid planning.

How to Guarantee Your Medicaid Payments on Day 101

You now know that Medicare fully covers your first 20 days in a nursing home and a smaller portion of nursing home cost after that, up to 100 days. This is what we consider our critical period. This is the period of time when we absolutely must begin to prepare for receiving Medicaid.

Hopefully some preparations have been made before this point in a client/patient's care. This is often not the case, but what we ideally want is for Medicaid to start picking up the cost beginning the day after Medicare coverage expires, often beginning the first day of the very next month after Medicare.

To do this, during the first 100 days under Medicare coverage we want to spend down the client/patient's assets to the average required maximum—in most states—of $2,000 in total assets for a non-married/widowed person. This allows us to qualify for Medicaid coverage by Day 101.

CHERYL L. FLETCHER-DOCHERTY

Obviously, the dollar value of assets you are allowed to keep, and the amount of assets that must be liquidated, depend entirely upon your state of care.

If you are married, those numbers change drastically. If you are married and have an at-home spouse, in most states and as of 2011 you were allowed to keep half of your *countable* assets up to $109,560. In 2012, this amount will increase to $113,640.

Some states use $109,560 as the *maximum* equation, citing the maximum amount of money your at-home spouse will be allowed to keep. Putting it another way, your at-home spouse will be able to keep the first $109,560 of your assets. After that, the remaining amount of assets must be spent down in order for you to qualify for Medicaid (states including California and Florida currently maintain the latter equation.)

Medicaid does permit a small resource allowance for the institutionalized spouse, which is normally around $2,000 a month (the amount depends upon the state you live in). Given this equation, married couples have a total of $111,560 as the maximum amount of funds they may have in their possession before spend-down would be required.

In states using the *minimum/maximum* equation, the stay-at-home spouse is able to keep half of the remaining assets, up to the maximum of $109,560. So, in order for the at-home spouse to keep $109,560, they have to have at least twice that amount, or $219,120—they have to have countable assets of $219,120 initially—in order to keep $109,560. That said, Medicaid will require a spend-down of the rest of your countable assets over and above the $109,560 unless we shift it over to income, which we normally do. Or, we can convert to some other asset Medicaid considers exempt.

Medicaid Exempt/Compliant Assets

Let's start with a very simple Medicaid-exempt asset strategy.

Let's assume that we have $100,000 belonging to Mr. Smith, who is in a nursing home and is allowed to keep $2,000. Unfortunately, and without a solid Medicaid plan, the other portion of his assets, or $98,000, must be spent down.

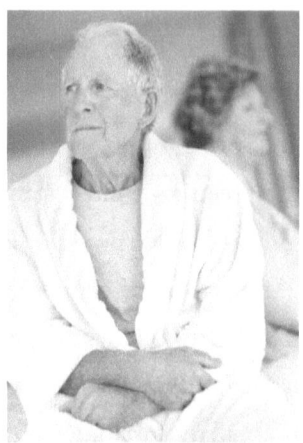

Fortunately, we have an alternative to this all-too-often last resort. We can convert that remaining $98,000 into an income stream for Mr. Smith. With this strategy, Medicaid no longer looks at the remaining $98,000 as a countable asset; they now see it as an income stream, and that income stream could be created through a Medicaid compliant annuity.

"Medicaid Compliant" Annuities

All sorts of insurance people are representing all kinds of annuities as being Medicaid compliant/friendly, but not all such annuities will pass the sniff test when it comes time to qualify for Medicaid.

Again, each state has different requirements regarding the precise definition of a so-called "Medicaid-compliant" annuity, which is why it is so important to seek expert advice when considering the purchase of any annuity for Medicaid planning purposes. You need to get it right or major problems can occur, and you will need a qualified Medicaid Planning Specialist to get it right.

First, the annuity must be permanently and totally "irrevocable." It must be "non-assignable." It must be "non-transferrable." It must contain "no cash value." It must also be "non-commutable," meaning that you cannot—at any time during that Medicaid recipient's lifetime—convert that annuity to cash. And only a very few companies provide such annuities. Although many companies say they do, they *do not*.

The truly Medicaid compliant annuity also must be "actuarially sound," meaning that it has to be set up to pay out during/within the Medicaid recipient's life expectancy. Depending upon the state, Medicaid officials have their own charts to determine a patient's life expectancy, and the annuity's pay-out schedule must adhere to the state's chart, in order for it to be Medicaid compliant.

If Medicaid officials determine that your annuity is Medicaid compliant, the principle within that annuity will be exempt from Medicaid spend-down.

Yet, as stated above, one state might require that the annuity adhere to a pay-out over a recipient's life expectancy while another state may allow a shorter payout period, within one's life expectancy. Each state is different, and each and every state will have exacting guidelines for their own specific terms of compliance. This is why the advice of a qualified specialist is so important in this area. Too many people assume they know every detail regarding compliance—some even think all states have the same compliance guidelines—but the vast majority representing compliant annuities fall short of having real knowledge and it will cost you dearly.

Too many financial planners simply do not know that an annuity's compliance may depend upon the payout provided by the annuity carrier. Some states, Idaho for example, go a bit further, saying that the annuity itself must provide a guaranteed 3.45% annual return, or better (for 2008). A 3.45% annual return?!

There are few to no annuities out there that will be truly Medicaid compliant AND pay out an impressive 3.45% return. Idaho therefore makes it virtually impossible to use annuities (without obtaining additional verifications) for Medicaid planning because Medicaid compliant annuities are not designed for growth, they are designed for protection.

In other states, the Medicaid annuity itself—even though compliant—isn't sufficient enough. We have to provide verification letters from the writing company itself confirming that the policy issued was indeed totally and permanently irrevocable, non-assignable, non-transferable, non-commutable and has no cash value. And in some states we have to take an extra step and provide refusal letters from companies (who are in the business of purchasing immediate annuities) showing that they are NOT able to purchase the annuity—in that it is non-assignable, non-transferable, and has no cash value, that it is a truly Medicaid compliant annuity.

Once again, we Medicaid Planning Specialists need to know precisely what kinds of annuities to provide on our end, in order to negate the kinds of objections that Medicaid case workers are likely to come up with. Otherwise, our Medicaid applications would never make it through the system.

Annuity Nightmares

Here's the basic problem with Medicaid compliant annuities: Medicaid case workers really have no idea which companies carry Medicaid compliant annuities. They are not in this business. So, they will instruct us, according to their state regulations, to provide support in the form of letters (applicable in some states) from two, maybe three, insurance carriers that are in the business of buying these types of annuities. Further, we will have to show that these types of annuities are truly non-assignable, non-transferrable, irrevocable and have no cash value because that annuity cannot be assigned, that payments from the annuity cannot be assigned, that the annuity was set up to be truly irrevocable and non-assignable so that we cannot change the beneficiary or the payee over to that annuity provider or anyone else.

Preying on desperate people who have purchased so-called compliant annuities that fail Medicaid standards, there are predatory insurance carriers (in my opinion) that are set up to buy annuities from individuals at a set percentage well below the annuity's actual cash value, thus providing the individual with immediate cash for spend-down. Yet, the same company leaves the individual vulnerable to other fees (I'll explain shortly).

Meanwhile, there are so many insurance agents out there who are selling improper annuities to a senior population trying to qualify for Medicaid. The agents do not want to lose the business so they sell them an improper annuity anyway and walk away—far away—with the commission.

Yes, the annuity they sell might qualify as an "immediate" annuity. It might even be irrevocable. Yet, because that annuity does not include important, additional language that Medicaid officials look for, it will NOT qualify. And that puts a senior at a financial disability, a financial hardship, because now they have this immediate annuity that is irrevocable—and they can't get out of it. The annuity turns out to be a TOTALLY COUNTABLE asset because it doesn't meet the definition of a Medicaid annuity.

This sort of situation turns my stomach because it should never have occurred. Not only that, but this class of agent muddies up the water for the rest of us, who are trying to make a positive difference in people's lives by utilizing proper products and techniques.

The senior might have initially been thinking that by going to a licensed insurance agent, the agent would automatically know which annuities qualify for Medicaid. Unfortunately, a great many agents have no clue as to the real specifics of Medicaid compliance. Sure, they may have heard that annuities work for protecting assets from Medicaid spend-down, but they have to be set up in proper form. So, the insurance agent sells the senior an annuity. Later, the senior tries to qualify for Medicaid, and Medicaid says, "We're sorry but your annuity doesn't qualify. You converted your $100,000 CD over to this annuity, which is assignable. Therefore, we deem the annuity to be a non-exempt asset which is entirely countable."

All along, the senior has been told that only the income stream from the immediate annuity would be countable to Medicaid. Now the senior finds that Medicaid will count the whole enchilada. Given the senior's possession of the countable, irrevocable $100,000 annuity, it would take years for the senior to qualify for Medicaid. How will she cash out the principal if it is irrevocable? And if the company does allow cash-out, the surrender penalties will be immense. Yet most companies won't even cash out because the annuity is irrevocable. Catch 22. What now?

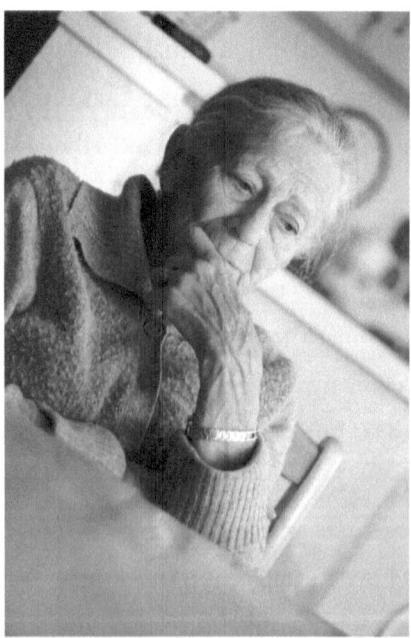

Her only option is to ideally have wealthy family members who can buy her out and assign the income stream to themselves, or to approach one of those predatory annuity purchasers mentioned above. While irrevocable, the annuity is assignable (the latter being a disqualifying factor for Medicaid). The senior now goes to the purchasing company hat-in-hand and asks, "What will you give me? I need out." The basic answer: The $100,000 annuity that she just purchased is now worth 50 cents on the dollar. If she assigns the scheduled $100,000 worth of annuity payments over to the company, the company will give her $50,000 right then in exchange.

The hapless senior may now take her remaining $50,000—after losing $50,000—and go out and buy a properly structured Medicaid annuity. But here's the real kick in the pants: While the senior has already lost half of the value of her annuity to the purchasing company, Medicaid sees only that she just sold an annuity worth $100,000 for less than fair market value. MEDICAID IS GOING TO PENALIZE HER FOR THAT!

Medicaid may even penalize the senior for the amount of money she lost against fair-market value because, according to Medicaid thinking, Mrs. Smith dumped her annuity as a Medicaid solution. Look at it this way, the original $100,000 value of the annuity would have been countable for Medicaid spend-down, right? Well, now it isn't, and the resulting Medicaid penalty could be stiff, up to, say, 20% of the original $100,000 principal, which now must come out of the remaining $50,000 our hapless senior just received from the purchasing carrier.

In the end, and through improper Medicaid planning, our senior walks away from the deal with only $30,000 out of the original $100,000.

That is financially devastating. I get a lot of people coming to me after the fact with this type of situation in hand, a situation no one can afford.

Again, it is very, very important to have this sort of thing done properly. Too many people in the insurance business know a little bit about a subject with myriad twists and turns, yet they think they know it all. Well, they might know that the annuity must be non-commutable, but do they know that it must also be actuarially sound according to individual state guidelines? Maybe, maybe not. In the end, they get a nice commission for the sale of the annuity and the senior gets the shaft.

In fact, many of the Medicaid annuity companies will not make the annuity irrevocable in every way unless we press them to do it, and we must indicate our preference in writing. Meanwhile, some states require that irrevocable beneficiaries be named on the contract, and they must be specifically named as "irrevocable" beneficiaries. The contract itself may be irrevocable, but it might leave room for someone to go in later and change beneficiary designations, therefore making the contract in some way revocable. Meaning: you can't get out of the contract itself but you can make minor changes within it. Medicaid then says NO, not in any way shape or form are you allowed to meddle with that contract, so the contract is accordingly deemed "non-compliant." The application is denied, thanks to an incompetent Medicaid planner.

Further, all states adhering to the federal Deficit Reduction Act of 2005 now require that the state be named beneficiary, in some position, in a Medicaid compliant annuity. At this writing, all but two states in America adhere to the DRA.

If you are married, the state may take a back-seat beneficiary position to the spouse, but if you are not married, the state may require that it be in the first beneficiary position in your annuity. Putting it another way, if you are fortunate enough to be married, Medicaid may take a contingency position as beneficiary of the Medicaid compliant annuity. This means that the spouse gets the annuity if you pass away and Medicaid gets nothing—IF the annuity qualifies.

I accordingly get a lot of contacts from lawyers who have me go over their client annuity contracts to make certain that they comply with every detail required by a particular state. Georgia, for example, may have its own specific rules, while another state may very only slightly, but all it takes is one call from the Medicaid case worker assigned to your Medicaid application to raise a flag. Your annuity must be iron-clad compliant because once you make that purchase, it's set in stone, and unless it is done just-so, you are not going to qualify for Medicaid.

Dealing With Social Security and Pensions

I can't call Social Security and ask them to stop sending you checks. I can't call companies sending pension checks and stop them, either. If I were able to do that, Medicaid would step forward and point out that I was the lawful owner of that income. Even if I chose not to receive it, they would count it against me.

In mainstream Medicaid planning, Social Security will be paid out to whomever it is due and that kind of income—including pension income—does need to go toward the cost of care in the nursing home.

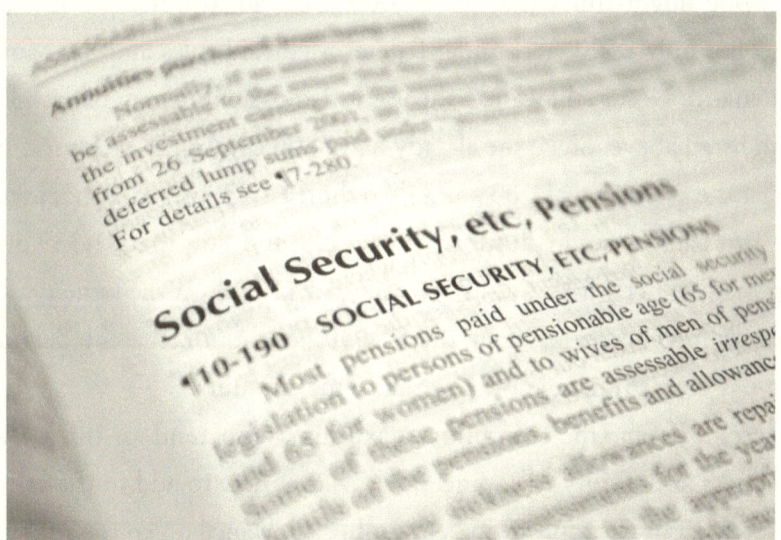

However, if you have a community spouse, there is a way to create a shifting of income. For example, if the community spouse is a female, she might have a lower Social Security payment since she earned less during her working years. Or, she might be receiving the Social Security minimum payment. In this case, all states allow for a Monthly Maintenance Needs Allowance and most states allow a minimum and maximum allowance. The minimum for most states in 2011 was $1,839 and the maximum was $2,739; the maximum will be $2,841 in 2012.

In those states that have the minimum/maximum allowance, there is also a Shelter and Utility Allowance that can be utilized in an effort to obtain a higher Monthly Maintenance Needs Allowance.

Many financial planners and insurance agents don't know it but a solution exists with this little nugget. Let's say the female spouse in this scenario is receiving only $500 a month in Social Security, while the husband in the nursing home is receiving Social Security and a pension with a combined total of $3,000. When both were living at home, their combined $3,500 was sufficient to live comfortably. But now that he's living in the nursing home, one might think that his $3,000 must go to nursing home costs, leaving her only $500. Yet, under federal Medicaid rules and the Monthly Maintenance Needs Allowance, she is entitled to a minimum of $1,839 per month listed above. Since she already had $500 coming in each month, we subtract the $500 from $1,839 and she's short $1,339 per month. However, we can go back to her institutionalized spouse and shift that $1,339 over to her, providing her with a monthly income of $1,839. At the same time, her husband's income decreases by the $1,339 per month, thereby decreasing his co-pay to the nursing home by that same amount.

States offering the minimum/maximums also tend to offer Shelter Allowances and Utility Allowances, which are there to add to the at-home spouse's $1,839 per month, increasing her allowance up to the maximum of $2,739—if possible.

And maybe there's a monthly mortgage payment. Maybe she's in an assisted living program and paying a monthly payment to that facility.

Maybe she's paying rent. Whatever she is paying could be considered an extra shelter allowance. So, we take those expenses and utility expenses, real estate taxes, condo or co-op maintenance fees, and her home owner's insurance and try—according to individual state equations—to get her up to that $2,739.

With pensions, such equations are true as well. Pensions must remain in the true owner's name. If Mary, who is living at home, has only $500 of her own Social Security, her husband's pension and Social Security income may be incorporated, combined and shifted in the same way, to give Mary the same kind of outcome under the state's Monthly Maintenance Needs Allowances.

Home Health Care and Other Issues

Maybe Mary is living at home but has her own health care issues to deal with. Medicaid refers to this as "living in the community" and Mary may be eligible for Medicaid to pay for certain services if she qualifies. This is possible through a program is known as "Home and Community Based Services" or "HCBS".

Home and Community Based Services, in general, will pay for personal care services including dressing, bathing, cooking, cleaning, grocery shopping and the rest. Even some levels of respite care are included. Respite care applies when a patient is placed in a nursing home for a few days to give the caregiver a break, or if the home patient gets sick and needs hospitalization.

Also included in home-based services are adult day care, medications, oxygen, walking the dog and "habilitation"—meaning, to assist someone to improve their mobility, help with financial management, hygiene—all those things required to get them back to normal.

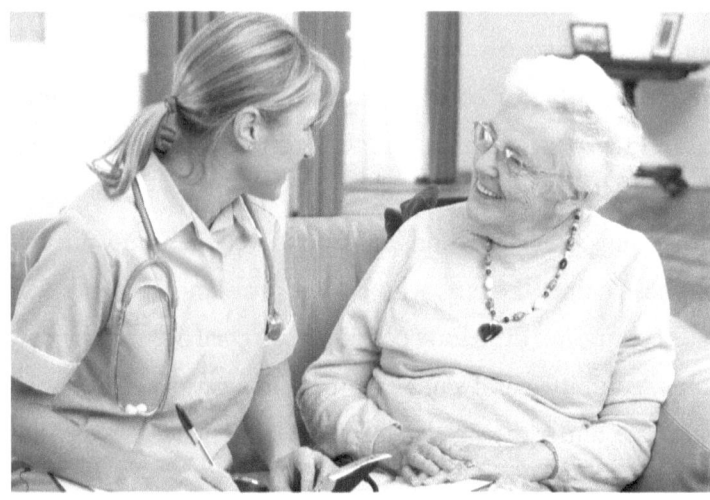

Another category often overlooked is case management. Case managers ensure that the right care providers are assigned to the home. They are basically paid to review, manage and supervise a patient's care, or challenge the quality of care giving, if necessary.

Some Medicaid-certified Assisted Living centers can handle Medicaid patients. But you MUST know in advance if your chosen facility is properly certified.

Go to MEDICARE.GOV to find out if your chosen state or county facility is either Medicare and/or Medicaid certified. And while Assisted Living is the place to begin for many heading for Medicaid—even before Medicare is required—this can be the time to initiate Medicaid spend-down and other advance planning measures.

In one case, a 73-year-old woman entered the assisted living system and remained in assisted living for more than five years before she had a change of health requiring nursing home care. The previous five-year period would have been ideal for protecting the remaining $30,000 in her bank account from Medicaid.

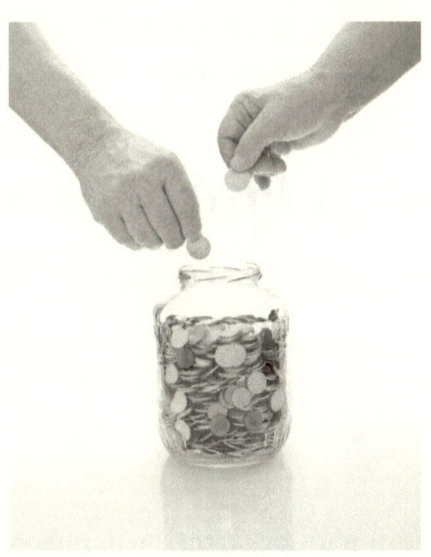

So, even the smallest amounts are worth protecting and there are no minimum amounts for Medicaid planning, but the longer you hold out the more it will cost you. In this case, assuming she was eligible for Medicaid, we would have taken $28,000 and converted over to something Medicaid compliant, probably a Medicaid annuity, leaving $2,000 in her bank account for the Medicaid minimum of allowable, countable assets.

Either way, unless you know what to do, you will end up spending everything on your cost of care. Medicaid will exempt a burial plan, for example, although there are limitations to the cost and you should be aware of spending caps in each state. Also, burial plans should be iron-clad irrevocable. But with the rest of her money, while living in the assisted living center she could purchase better furniture, a plasma TV and even a new automobile. While in a nursing home, one vehicle can be exempt and given to an heir at a later time (after death), although vehicle values have caps as well, in some states.

As always, the five-year look-back period under Medicaid must be considered when gifting, which is a gamble in this situation.

CHAPTER 3

Critical Problems with LTC Coverage and Trusts

"Look-Back" Periods and Penalty Extensions

I F YOU HAVE private long term care insurance, what people often fail to consider is that the former look-back period under Medicaid was once only a three-year period of time.

The "look back" period is a period of time when Medicaid looks at everything you own and everything you gifted or transferred to anyone. Anything found during the look-back period is considered part of your Medicaid spend-down requirement. Again, the old look-back period began the day you made the gift or transfer.

But Congress suddenly changed the rules. Now, we face a five-year look-back period and that applies to every state that adopted the Deficit Reduction Act of 2005. Those states include all but two—Illinois and California—both of which are soon to adopt the DRA.

Before moving on, the dilemma created by a simple extension of the look-back period point to a glaring necessity. In this era, when proposed changes of entitlement programs loom at every turn of the political mile, you will definitely need to have your Medicaid planning strategy periodically reviewed.

Getting back to recent changes that have upended many a Medicaid planning strategy, again it is critical to note that federal Medicaid rules now require a **five-year** look-back period. The five year look-back period commences on the date you apply for Medicaid. Anything gifted or transferred within this five-year period will be considered part of the amount you personally owe the nursing home under Medicaid. If you lack the money to cover the cost of what you gifted or transferred during the five-year look-back period, Medicaid calculations will add the value of those gifts and transfers and render a "penalty period." This penalty period equates to an extended delay of your Medicaid benefits, which will be equal in dollar value to the amount you gifted or transferred during the five-year look-back period. This often measures in coverage delays of many months or even years, during which you would be required to pay for nursing home costs out of your own pocket.

There are companies that will write additional, supplemental long term care coverage for people in older age categories, but they have to clear underwriting, which depends on their health status. Not only that, can they afford additional coverage that has become prohibitively expensive as we age?

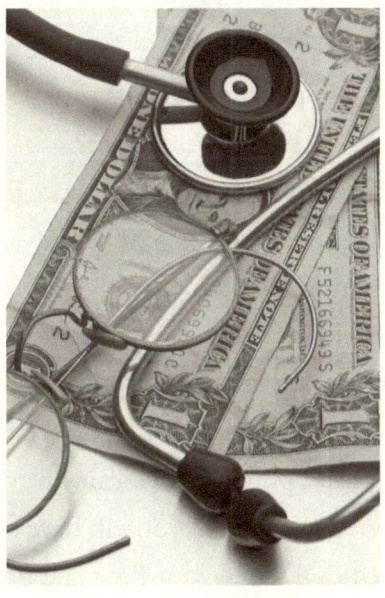

Problems Related to "Look-Back" and LTC Insurance

The change in the federal look-back period from three to five years has indeed caused significant problems for people holding certain Long Term Care insurance policies. If you are in this situation you should consult a Medicaid Planning Specialist to address problems facing a host of policy holders.

Before changes in the federal look-back period went into effect, all financial planning practitioners thought the same thing: Provide enough nursing home insurance to cover the three-year Medicaid look-back period so we could do all of the appropriate Medicaid planning necessary to get everything out of a client's name—within the three-year look-back period.

All sorts of people accordingly bought long term care insurance with three years of coverage in mind. In addition, many weren't savvy enough, or appropriately advised, to buy coverage with an added inflation factor in the policy. Instead, they purchased long term care policies that provided the one-time going rate of $100 per day for care in a nursing home and the policy would expire after three years.

As time went by, you might have paid off your policy, expecting it to do what it's supposed to do—cover the three-year gap. Ten years later, you're in a nursing home and your private long-term-care insurance kicks in. Yet, now the average nursing home cost is $200 a day and Medicaid requires a five-year look-back period. So, you are only half-covered for three years and fully exposed to asset reduction for another two, full years.

As for the difference between your policy coverage and increased nursing home costs, you can go ahead and pay the difference out of your own pocket, OR, you can apply for Medicaid to pick up the difference! That's right: Under certain conditions you can have both private long-term care insurance and Medicaid coverage at the same time.

Most people don't know that. Most people use their policy until it's all used up, and then they try to qualify for Medicaid, but *there are ways to do both at the same time.*

Another option would be to purchase a tax-deferred annuity with a long term care rider. If 50% of the policy remains deferred in its accumulation phase, the other 50% can be paid out without penalty for long term care, but we'll address annuities—*and their limitations*—in later chapters.

Trusts: Irrevocable and Otherwise

If you actually want to protect your money from Medicaid spend-down, we would need to do some Medicaid planning well in advance. The younger you are and the earlier you get started, the more we can protect your money. But people don't like to do that. They don't like to give up control of their assets. Yet, if you are going to protect everything, this would be necessary. You would have to title your house—literally give it away—into an irrevocable trust, or give it to your children prior the five year look-back window. To really envelope your holdings in a sound citadel of financial planning, you can literally give your assets away in such a trust, but the 70-plus age group doesn't like to do that. I mean, can you find a family member to be named as a trust beneficiary that you can trust to give those assets back to you, if and when you need them?

Perils of the "Revocable/Irrevocable" Trust

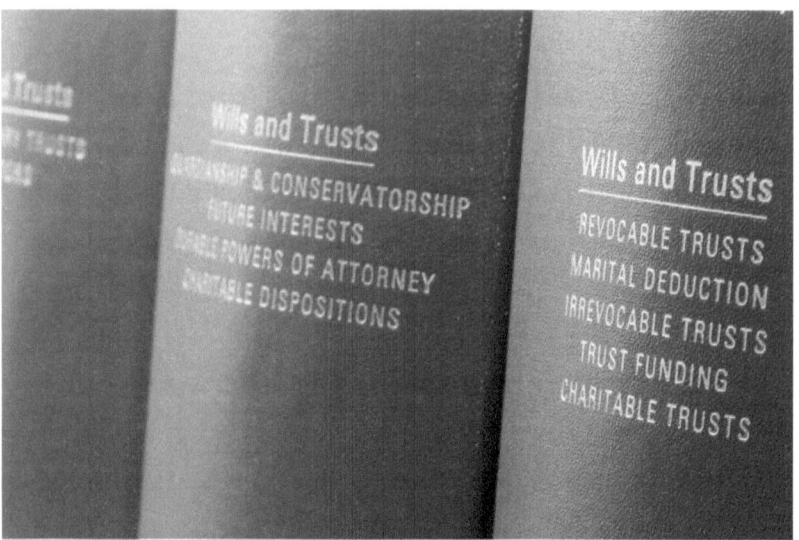

A "revocable" trust—meaning, a trust that can be changed or revoked—unfortunately won't work with Medicaid, which considers the revocable trust an available asset. It is available because the trust is revocable, right? You have every right to revoke the trust and have access to anything in the trust, which exposes anything funding the trust as an asset subject to Medicaid spend-down. For example, a vehicle normally deemed to be excluded would be considered countable if it were transferred into a trust.

The problem with an "irrevocable" trust—meaning, a trust that *cannot* be changed or revoked—is that, in the case of transferring assets into the trust, those transfers, if they cannot be distributed back to you under any circumstance, would be considered a gift. If any of the assets which are transferred to the trust are available to be distributed back to you, that amount available to you would be considered a countable asset for Medicaid purposes. And the rest, if any, would be considered a gift, which is subject to a penalty if made within the five year look-back period.

The obvious solution is to have set-up the trust well enough in advance so that the five year look-back period has expired. The transfers made to the trust are no longer deemed as countable assets, no matter what their value may be.

In this situation and many others, always consult an elder law or Medicaid-savvy attorney who is well familiar with rules within your state. Your Medicaid Planning Specialist may have a directory of such individuals as well.

CHAPTER 4

True Stories . . . from Medicaid Hades

I F YOU STILL have any doubts about seeking help with your Medicaid planning, the following are a few sanity-saving reasons why an objective, third-party Medicaid advocate should be in your corner whenever you approach Medicaid—be it in the initial application process, or during one of many critical-care transitions along the way.

In this chapter, I show you living examples, from my own archives, of the ways a Medicaid Planning Specialist can cut through the monumental heaps of bureaucratic red tape and swarms of conflicting rules and regulations. I'll even show you a few little known rules and regulations people working inside the Medicaid system have ever heard of!

All told, knowing more about how the system works will help you understand why applications and procedural problems sometimes occur. When you understand the root of the problem, solutions suddenly begin to appear as if some dense, invisible curtain had been removed, making the life easier for patients and care-giving family members.

Know Your Case Worker

A typical scenario would be greatly alleviated, for example, by simply knowing the case worker assigned to your case, also knowing where to submit certain types of applications and when. In some states, you have no choice in determining which way the process will go. Your case is simply handed off to someone in the Medicaid system and your application or appeal may be at the mercy of that person. Yet, even in those cases, I would try to walk the case worker through each step of your case. Unfortunately, most lay-people, including dedicated family members, wouldn't know how to do that because they wouldn't know what a case worker is looking for. Even if they have some information, the process is just too cumbersome, the volume of information too great.

Here, however, are a few things that Medicaid case workers will look for in your application:

Assets vs. Income: Many times people list these in the wrong columns, especially when it comes to listing an annuity (a properly structured Medicaid compliant annuity). Many inaccurately place the annuity under the Asset/Resource column and the caseworker is quick to include that in the client's countable resources. This causes the client to be falsely over-resourced when, in fact, the annuity should have been listed under the Income column, and then ONLY included as monthly income to the nursing home resident or, in some cases, his or her spouse.

Some caseworkers do not allocate the income appropriately, especially annuity income. Some automatically allocate the annuity income to the nursing home resident, increasing his or her nursing home co-pay and minimizing the income that is rightfully owned by the community spouse. In some cases, if the total income exceeds the nursing home private pay rate, this would create an error that would disqualify the nursing home resident from receiving Medicaid benefits.

Caseworkers want to make certain that all proofs and verifications are provided for every line of the Medicaid application for which you provide information or responses. This often includes five years of statements for each and every account you own/owned individually or jointly. It also includes an explanation of all transfers and gifts made, along with verification of amounts and dates to which they were made.

If you do not supply caseworkers with all information they request, your case will be denied due to your failure to provide them with the information.

In those states that have an "income limit/cap" for the nursing home resident, some caseworkers will deny eligibility if the resident is over the cap, without advising them that a special kind of trust is needed and would fix the issue.

Knowing all of the above and more, if I can get in touch with that case worker and work directly, one-on-one, with that person in order to have everything done "just-so," according to the way they need to have things done, situations can change dramatically in favor of my clients. Connections help, of course, as in any business. Through the years, I've been able to get to know a great many Medicaid case workers across the nation and one contact leads to another.

Based on my level of experience with case workers, I do need to be frank with you about one reality, a basic, human reality that applies everywhere we go in life: *Some case workers are going to be more diligent than others*, and that's a fact. These people are not machines. They are human beings with a tough job to do and they all have their individual ways of looking at, and dealing with, your situation.

While this sounds like simple information, it's a very important perspective to have when approaching Medicaid. Simply put, some case workers are far more strict than others when it comes to adhering to every letter of jurisdictional rules and regs.

Another harsh reality: There are indeed some Medicaid case workers who believe that virtually no one should be able to obtain Medicaid coverage! They might have been immersed in anti-entitlement-program political rhetoric for a long time. Who knows? What matters is that you know about some of the challenges I face every day. Putting a human face in

Forest Gump's box of chocolates, 'you never know who you're going to get.' Armed with this knowledge, imagine what can happen to the completely uninitiated lay person entering the system for the first time!

Contentious Case Workers

This is especially true when you have just converted a Certificate of Deposit worth over $100,000 into something like a Medicaid-compliant annuity. Some case workers don't like it! They will try to fight you, using every possible trick and tactic to disqualify that annuity.

But if they fight with me, they're going to lose because I know how to counter their objections AND I know precisely how to make sure that annuity will ensure iron-clad qualification. Armed with the right knowledge, you need not fear receiving objections from Medicaid case workers. So often, you will encounter a case worker who doesn't know her own state rules, which means that YOU must be able to provide solid, documented proof to back up any argument you propose.

This means that you will have to know well in advance where to get that proof—based on their own state Medicaid statutes—and where to get it quickly in some situations. You must be able to fight back when they throw objections at you—with their own state statutes. You must be able to say to a case worker: "You might be trying to tell me it's this way, but I am going to tell you that your own state regulation states otherwise," and you must be able to back it up with proof from their own state manuals/archives.

I just went through this with the State of Missouri, for example. We were dealing with a Medicaid compliant annuity, and I had to prove to them that the annuity was truly compliant within their own state Medicaid rules and regulations. One of the requirements demands that the state be named as a beneficiary of the annuity. The nature of the state's position as a beneficiary depends upon the nature of your *marital status*. This case involved a community spouse, so I was able to name the state as a contingent beneficiary. But the case worker had other ideas; she was convinced that the state had to be named as the primary beneficiary, which is not true. In fact, it is clearly stated in black and white (as of this printing) that if a community spouse exists, the state will be named as a *contingent* beneficiary, which is a HUGE difference. It means that if the annuity owner/Medicaid recipient dies in a nursing home, the community spouse will get to keep all of the remaining principle in the annuity.

Knowing this, I still had to argue our case. I had to go back and find the regulation and put it directly in front of the case worker. Yet, after I got that one past her, she came back to me and said "this application still doesn't qualify." I asked, "Well, why not?" She answered, "The way you have the beneficiary designation worded on the annuity application won't work for us. We want you to name the State of Missouri as the beneficiary 'to the extent of any benefits paid on behalf of the specific name of the annuity owner/Medicaid applicant'" who would eventually become the Medicaid recipient. I had used the term "Medicaid recipient" instead of using the recipient's actual name, which was perfectly valid since the recipient's name was clearly stated throughout the annuity documents in question. We all knew who the Medicaid recipient was in this case; the application had been filed, the recipient clearly named. But the case worker kept arguing with me on this one, small point.

The point here is that such a miniscule, niggling detail can easily derail your Medicaid application, and you may never know it. You would simply receive a notice of application denial.

In situations where I encounter a point of impasse with a case worker, I finally go for some kind of recourse, such as asking for the intervention of a supervisor.

Since we don't want to alienate the person we've been working with before resorting to her supervisor, this can make for rough sailing in the social-political sense of the word. Remember, the case worker, the person we've been dealing with, has not left the building. She may be working feverishly, in fact, to defend her own position by trying to disqualify your case, which can obviously cause problems if your case goes to review. So, demanding to move up the food chain and speak with a supervisor must be done with care, and only when absolutely appropriate. Putting it another way, you must never jump up and throw a fit when things aren't going your way, immediately demanding to speak to a supervisor. This is seen as fairly common behavior among those assisting disgruntled Medicaid applicants and will get you nowhere unless the timing and situation are just right.

I go to a supervisor or director *only* when I know I'm going to get an application denial and that the denial will not be legitimate according to clearly stated rules and regulations. Putting it another way, if I know that the case worker is absolutely in the wrong and fails to recognize that fact or offer their cooperation, I will then have enough ammunition to *demand* that our case go to a higher authority, and when I do this I am no longer concerned over the case worker because I know that they were going to deny it anyway.

Should the case worker and their supervisor not see eye-to-eye with me, and proceed to hand down a denial, it is at this time I request a sort of last-resort event the Medicaid system calls "Fair Hearing," but in this situation, what do we have to lose? Nothing. And in this situation, we are able to overturn the caseworker's decision, in that we are provided the opportunity to present our documentation and support to an outside, third party.

I would rather not put the client through what is called "Fair Hearing," which is where we're going in this type of case.

Fair Hearing occurs when Medicaid caseworkers either don't like your case, or you were declared ineligible because your financial situation appeared to them to exceed certain limitations. Or, they might be convinced that you transferred money improperly, or they might dislike your application for some other reason, and there are many.

Keep in mind that without knowing what you now know, a case worker can simply deny your application even if you were totally eligible, and you would never know the difference! It's crazy, but things like this happen. You've met every requirement, satisfied all of it, but since the case worker was just green or blatantly misinformed, you have to file for a Fair Hearing.

If this happens to you, it is high time—time long overdue—to bring in a professional Medicaid specialist because the "fair hearing" is not controlled by the time-tested boundaries of true legal proceedings in a real courtroom, some of which have been centuries in the making to ensure fair treatment for both sides of the argument.

The Fair Hearing is not even held in a court room in many states, which sounds good at first. It is just an apparently informal meeting, which is usually held in a spare room at your local Medicaid office. It is conducted before a fair hearing officer, who may or may not be an attorney, and the fair hearing officer can only rule on whether or not the department followed the rules. The officer cannot change the department rules.

At the Fair Hearing, you have the right to state your case and present your documentation. You have the right to testify on your own behalf, call witnesses, and cross examine any of the state's witnesses. You also have the right to be represented by an advocate or an attorney.

The next step, if we do not win at the Fair Hearing level, is to appeal the decision through your state court system. Depending on your state, some systems offer agency appeals directly to the highest state court, while others provide intermediate levels of appeal. If the issues of the case are significant enough, it may be advisable or most appropriate to seek action in a federal court.

As you can see, this road can become rather long, cumbersome, and costly. To avoid this, I like to try to go through whomever I can at a lower level before a final decision is rendered. Thus, before even applying for Fair Hearing, I like to re-present my entire case with all documentation clearly marked and accompanied by our points of contention. So much of the time, the proper presentation of a logical argument backed by good documentation can avert an escalated situation. This is especially true in advance, or during, Fair Hearing because the Fair Hearing Officer has the power to overturn decisions made at lower levels in the Medicaid hierarchy.

Processing the Medicaid Annuity

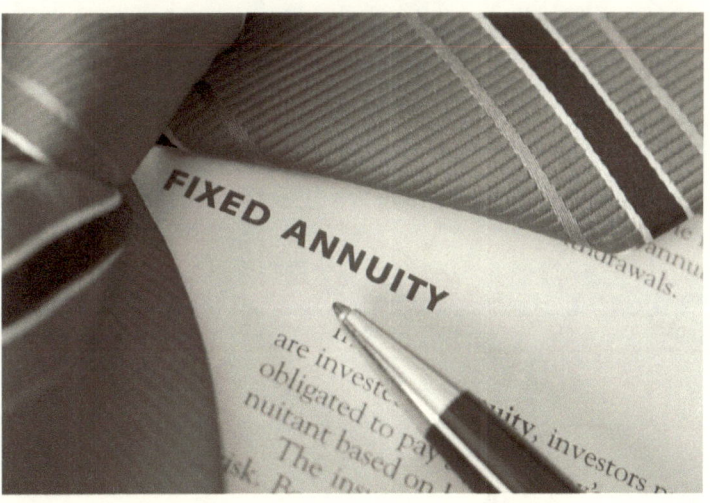

In this vein, you should know that your so-called Medicaid-compliant annuity will probably go straight to the top for review . . . at the very beginning stage of the application process. When Medicaid applications involve Medicaid compliant annuities, it is Medicaid procedure in many states that the individual annuity involved in your case would be sent to the top echelon of state Medicaid administration for careful study.

In some states, every single annuity being proposed with an application must be reviewed by the state. This is a big job involving reams of annuity contracts and mistakes can be made. Do state Medicaid officials always get it right? No, and this is precisely why you need a pro on your team before things have the first chance to unravel with a Medicaid application involving annuities.

Now that you have had a first-hand look at "real-life" procedural nightmares in the Medicaid system, let's address some of the many, misconceptions related to Medicaid:

CHERYL L. FLETCHER-DOCHERTY

CHAPTER 5

Notorious
Misconceptions

Misconception #1
Hiding money

S OME PEOPLE BELIEVE that they can just hide their money from Medicaid investigators, after the investigators have been assigned to examine a Medicaid application. People think, for example, that they can take money out of one of their bank accounts, hide the money under a mattress and be perfectly safe from scrutiny.

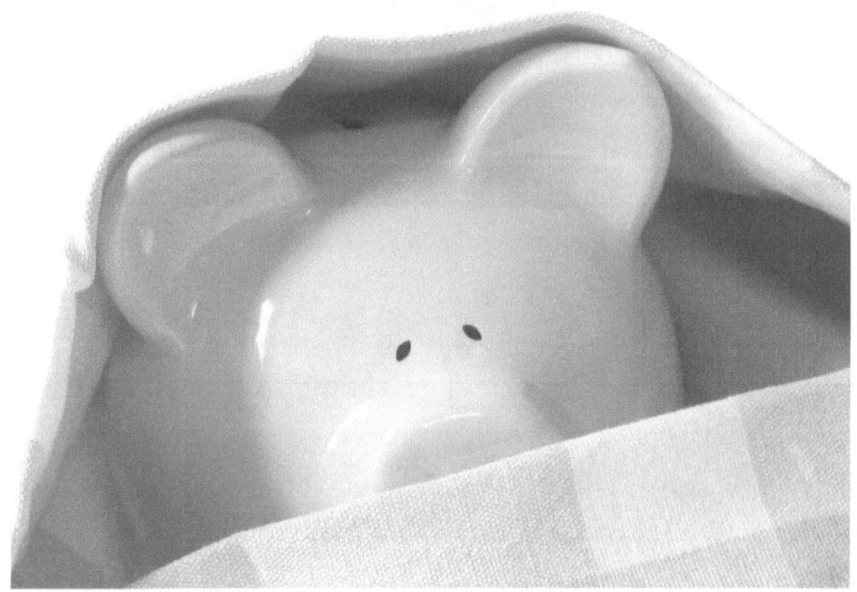

This won't work for obvious reasons. For one, we all know how easy it has become for the average computer hacker to uncover boatloads of financial information about virtually anyone. Do you think a highly skilled law enforcement official, like the typically Medicaid investigator, would be any less qualified to dig up information about you, especially when armed with all sorts of legal license to demand information from your banks and credit card companies?

Be absolutely certain of the fact that when you apply for coverage under Medicaid, you will be required to sign legal forms allowing Medicaid investigators to inspect every type of financial record related to you and your money.

Again, when you apply for Medicaid, today, you also face a five-year "look-back" period, during which Medicaid investigators literally look back at every banking transaction you have ever made during the past five-year period. They are also highly skilled at finding transactions you have made through other easily accessible records, which reveal a host of other financially related transactions you might have made during the same five-year look-back period, including the transfer of property titles, liquidation of real estate, the sale of stocks, bonds, mutual funds and virtually every other kind of transaction you can think of.

Keep in mind that Medicaid personnel in your state are highly skilled at conducting thorough financial research. Medicaid researchers are dedicated to the task of discovering financial transactions that would *disqualify* you from receiving Medicaid coverage.

That's right, they are not generally interested in approving your application unless you are deemed genuinely, legally poor, because this program was designed to serve the poor: the financially destitute, and children from poor families. It was never meant to serve wealthy people hoping to reap the benefits of the Medicaid system while preserving their own assets.

For those reasons and more, Medicaid officials will demand to see receipts for everything. If you withdrew money on a certain date, they will ask to see written proof of where the money went: Was it spent on medical care, groceries, or a trip to the moon? If the money was used for spend-down in a nursing home or for other legitimate items allowed under Medicaid regulations, you will be asked to provide proof during the five-year look-back period.

If you cannot provide such proof, they will naturally assume that you still have the money or that you have improperly transferred it away. They will ask you to reveal the location of that money. Your Medicaid case worker will say, "You've got it, so where is it?" And if you decline to reveal the location of the missing money, they will deny your Medicaid application and they have every right to do so.

What about stocks, bonds and overseas funds laundered through foreign accounts? I'm sure people try to get away with things like that, but when you apply for Medicaid you are actually signing a legal affidavit attesting to the fact that you have made full disclosure regarding the location of every penny of your assets. To do otherwise is fraud, pure and simple, and it would be fraud committed against your state and federal governments. Putting it another way, Medicaid fraud is serious business. You can be convicted of Medicaid fraud and the consequences may be rather severe. Investigations into suspected cases are pursued with the assistance of many federal and state-level agencies, including the FBI, the Department of Justice, and the Department of Health and Human Services. Penalties differ, based upon the amount of money siphoned out of federal and state Medicaid coffers, but imprisonment can extend well beyond a year, with additional fines attached for aggravating circumstances.

Misconception #2
I must cancel my existing health care coverage to qualify for Medicaid:

Completely false! Of course you can keep your current health care plan and I recommend that my clients do so, as long as possible. Any supplemental insurance that would cover things not covered by Medicaid will be greatly helpful, such as additional coverage for prescription drugs.

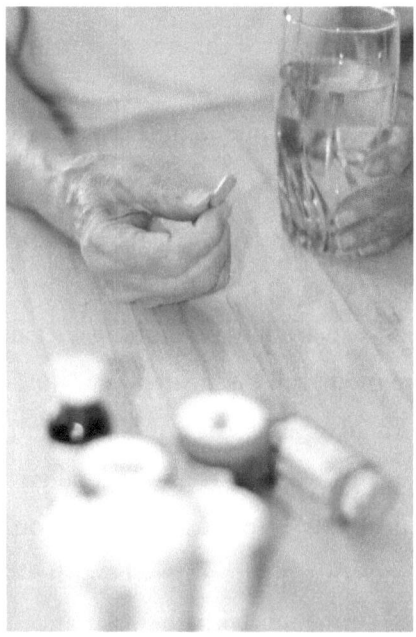

Your supplemental health care insurance policy also may provide additional coverage for cancer treatments not covered by Medicaid. So, having extra coverage for health care above and beyond Medicaid can be important when it comes to certain types of chemotherapy, radiation and other treatments.

Bottom line: Medicaid coverage may be limited when it comes to critically important care, so I do recommend that people keep their supplemental health care coverage as long as possible.

Whenever I devise a Medicaid plan for one of my clients, I will keep their existing health care policy in force because there are no good reasons to get rid of it AND because Medicaid not only allows you to have it, *they let you deduct the monthly cost of your supplemental health policy* right off the top of your monthly obligation to the nursing home.

For example, after allowable asset transfers have been made between, say, a wife living at home and her husband living in the nursing home, if the nursing home spouse is left owing, say, $1,000 a month to the nursing home, that amount would be reduced by the monthly premium owed for his supplemental health coverage, which can be considerable—more than $500 a month in some situations.

Of course, the cost of the at-home spouse's supplemental policy cannot be used to reduce her husband's spend-down obligation in the nursing home, but the advantages are obvious: She may have coverage for her own medical expenses under the supplemental policy, which she may need if she is both outside the Medicaid system and needs treatment not necessarily available under Medicare. Meanwhile, the husband in the nursing home would receive a spend-down deduction AND the assurance of coverage for certain treatments and prescriptions not covered by Medicaid.

Misconception #3
Medicaid/financial planning no longer apply to people in nursing homes

Wrong again. Medicaid planning can occur at any stage, even on the crisis side when someone is stricken with catastrophic illness in a nursing home. Take the case of a woman in a nursing home: She thinks that because she's in there, nothing else can happen and that she's all done. This is simply not true in most situations. You can always protect something.

We don't necessarily have all the options we once had, and more sophisticated strategies come into play when we have a widow or other non-married person in a nursing home because most legitimate asset transfers are allowable only between living spouses.

If you don't have a spouse and you come to me for help late in the day, the planning options are fewer and often less beneficial. I can't just annuitize an annuity you already own, for example, and send all the income back to a community spouse. Yet, there *are* strategies available that can benefit not only the Medicaid recipient in the nursing home but potential heirs, if the right elements fall into place.

First, I can take money she might have sitting in, say, a $50,000 bank CD—which is counted as an asset subject to spend-down—and convert it to a Medicaid-compliant annuity, which could give her a stream of monthly income. Most people do not know that money left to spend-down in a bank CD could otherwise be preserved for a much longer period as an annuity-based income stream.

In this situation, monthly income from the annuity would still be counted as income and would go to the nursing home, but the money would be paid out to the nursing home in much smaller increments. This could be a good thing in certain situations, but let's first address the wrong situation to involve annuities in Medicaid planning: If she has a family history of longevity, and if she is in good health other than having Alzheimer's, converting to the annuity might not work because she would eventually spend-down the annuity through countless monthly annuity income payments made to the nursing home through the years. Bit by bit, the entire annuity would be consumed through the annuity monthly income stream, because the income would go entirely to nursing home co-pays.

Yet, if she goes into the nursing home with a severe health condition and her medical prognosis determines that she would probably not live long from that point forward—maybe another six months—Medicaid planning could have powerful benefits for a beneficiary.

In this situation, I would take the $50,000 that was in her checking account or bank CD and convert it to income through a Medicaid compliant annuity. Yes, the monthly income stream from the annuity would still go to the nursing home co-pay but, again, only in small increments.

Now let's look at the numbers:

Remember that by qualifying for Medicaid, she has already gone from the nursing home's most expensive private-pay status to Medicaid pay-rate status. Under Medicaid status, the nursing home bill has already dropped from the typical $7,500 a month to the amount Medicaid is willing to pay—perhaps $3,500 a month.

When we additionally convert bank assets to the Medicaid compliant annuity—let's say she receives $500 a month from the annuity as income—she might be additionally receiving $1,000 from Social Security and another $1,000 a month from a teacher's pension. All told, she would be receiving $2,500 a month of her own total income, which would be slated for spend-down and go to the nursing home. The $2,500 would go toward settling the monthly nursing home fee, which is the maximum $3,500 allowed by Medicaid. The remaining difference is, of course, $1,000.

Here's where the power of the Medicaid compliant annuity kicks in: After she dies—in this case six months after converting to the income annuity—the state is only allowed to go after the annuity to the extent of the $1,000 difference between her former $2,500 income and the $3,500 Medicaid payout to the nursing home. That's all they can get: $1,000 from the annuity for each month she received Medicaid benefits.

Since she died after only six months in the nursing home, her six, $500-per-month income payouts from the annuity totaled only $3,000, which went to the nursing home. Subtracting the additional $1,000 difference mentioned above, which came due to Medicaid after she died, the original $50,000 principal in her annuity would still amount to $41,000.

Since the former Medicaid recipient is now deceased and no longer requires Medicaid benefits, the remaining $41,000 in the annuity *can go to anyone*—family, friends, anyone. That's the beauty of using Medicaid compliant annuities, but ONLY in certain situations that follow prescribed criteria.

Again, and as stated repeatedly in this book, you MUST ensure that ALL state criteria for Medicaid compliant annuities have been met, and to the letter, which is no easy matter and requires, in my opinion, professional assistance from a Medicaid Planning Specialist.

Misconception #4
Revocable trusts protect assets from Medicaid

This notion is absolutely incorrect and will cost you dearly in Medicaid planning.

A revocable trust allows you to revoke the trust, period. It allows you to gain full access to all assets inside the trust, anytime you want.

If you didn't hear me the first time, here it is again: Any assets placed in such a trust can be taken out of the trust by the creator of the revocable trust, including an annuity, and the assets can be freely spent. Therefore, if a trust is revocable, the asset is considered countable by Medicaid and subject to spend-down requirements.

Hello?! Why is this so hard for some people to understand? Through the years, I have been routinely amazed by those who think they can "hide" assets from Medicaid in a revocable trust. Put yourself in the shoes of a Medicaid case worker charged with protecting Medicaid from abuse at the hands of people trying to hotwire the system. Would you approve a Medicaid application from someone trying to protect their assets inside a revocable trust? Of course not, because you can yank your assets beyond the reach of Medicaid anytime you wish.

Because you have a right to it and access to it, a revocable trust is most often worthless for Medicaid planning purposes, although there are certain, limited, circumstances where they do offer a benefit.

Yet, enduring opinions persist among a few remaining lawyers and financial planners who think this kind of trust will protect assets from Medicaid. I've seen it time and again: In the eyes of Medicaid officials, it makes no difference if the trust carries a different title, with differing names in the title, like "The Revocable Living Trust of Lillian Smith, dated thus-and-such." Forget it. No matter what you are told and by whomever, I have encountered far too many costly, even tragic, situations over the years when revocable trusts smacked into Medicaid application procedures, and/or post-application review.

Misconception #5
I can give away $13,000 yearly; it will be exempt from Medicaid spend-down

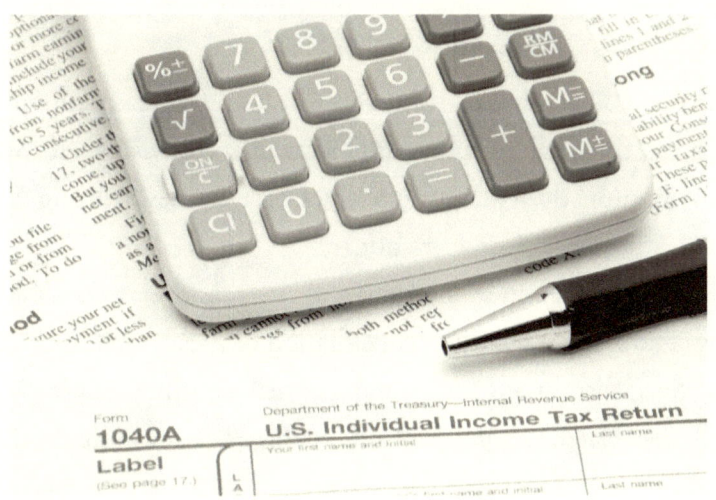

No way, and too many people get this confused with another exemption. The $13,000 exemption applies to the IRS and eligible IRS tax exemptions. People think that because the IRS is a federal agency and that Medicaid is essentially a federal program run by individual states, the $13,000 exemption applies to both entities. Where and how this erroneous notion got started is a mystery to me, but I have to re-explain the wheel on this one almost daily.

The short answer: your $13,000 IRS exemption has NOTHING to do with Medicaid.

Misconception #6
All annuities are created equal regarding Medicaid compliance

Are you kidding?

To be Medicaid compliant, each state has its own, often complicated set of specific criteria, some of which can be tricky and subject to individual interpretations among Medicaid case workers. Meaning: You must be ready to prove the compliance eligibility of your annuity through the presentation of supporting statutes, etc.

As strongly illustrated elsewhere in this book, a great many insurance sales people, financial planners and investment advisors are out there right now improperly representing scores of annuities as being Medicaid compliant, when they simply are not.

This is one of the most important and case-sensitive aspects of Medicaid planning. I strongly suggest the consultation of a truly qualified Medicaid Planning Specialist for anyone thinking of utilizing annuities for Medicaid strategies. See related chapters sections of this book for more details.

Misconception #7
All assets (IRAs, etc.) must be spent down prior to Medicaid acceptance

This is NOT true. These can be converted to Medicaid compliant instruments, following exacting guidelines, of course. Upon conversion and using the right vehicles, there are usually no immediate tax consequences. You are taxed only on the amount you take out of such vehicles in each calendar year.

Misconception #8
I can transfer real estate/other assets to kids and avoid Medicaid spend-down

Not unless you get started early in the game, which is precisely when you should get involved in Medicaid planning, even if you think you are healthy. If you wait too long, you will find yourself within Medicaid's federally mandated five-year look-back period. During this period, ANY asset transfers, including far-reaching categories from irrevocable trusts to stocks and bonds, will NOT be protected from Medicaid spend-down.

Misconception # 9
Any attorney/financial planner's estate protection plan protects against Medicaid spend-down

Not always. Elder planning and estate planning are quite a bit different, and they can differ from specific Medicaid planning strategies. Again, it's important to refer to a specialist before completing Medicaid planning strategies.

Plans should be checked for the presence of revocable trusts and even irrevocable trusts. For example, if your assets had been placed in an irrevocable trust more than five years prior to your Medicaid application, this would be perfect. If the irrevocable trust was created LESS than five years prior to the filing of your application, assets within the trust would be countable and subject to Medicaid spend-down. Please refer to the "trusts" section of this book for more details.

Misconception #10
Unreported assets escape spend-down because Medicaid cannot find them

This might sound comical to many, but you wouldn't believe how many people think this erroneous assumption applies to them. Of course they can find every nickel of your hidden assets! Please read this book for more information and become especially aware of the consequences of Medicaid fraud.

Misconception #11
If a spouse enters a nursing home, all of his/her assets go to the nursing home

This can happen, but only if you avoid good, professional Medicaid planning. There are ways to perform shifts of assets and income to provide additional monies for an at-home spouse, etc. You need not lose it all! You can, in most cases, retain a good deal of your assets.

Misconception #12
All nursing homes accept Medicaid patients

This is a very common misconception. NO, not all facilities accept Medicaid patients. In fact, many facilities that once accepted Medicaid no longer participate in the program. You need to ask up front, first and foremost, about a nursing home's relationship with Medicaid. Even though you may not be considering the use of Medicaid at the time, you might later on.

There are available directories listing active Medicaid nursing homes and assisted living centers in your area, which are mentioned elsewhere in this book.

Misconception #13
All assets can be discovered by Medicaid

Not necessarily. Non-liquid assets lacking a paper trail may include inherited art work including paintings and sculptures. Other assets in this group might include baseball card collections, gold and even collectables including ceramics and other items.

The dilemma begins after such items are sold and the proceeds are placed in track-able bank accounts, financial instruments, real estate, etc. Timing is critical when marketing such assets if they are to be counted within the estate of a potential Medicaid beneficiary.

CHAPTER 6

Applying for Medicaid . . . Avoiding Costly Errors

THIS CHAPTER ADDRESSES the basic steps needed to apply for Medicaid, which may come in handy if we find ourselves emotionally stressed and looking for guidance.

First, go to the local county Medicaid office (often referred to as the Department of Human Services, or Department of Social Services, etc.) where you want to apply for Medicaid.

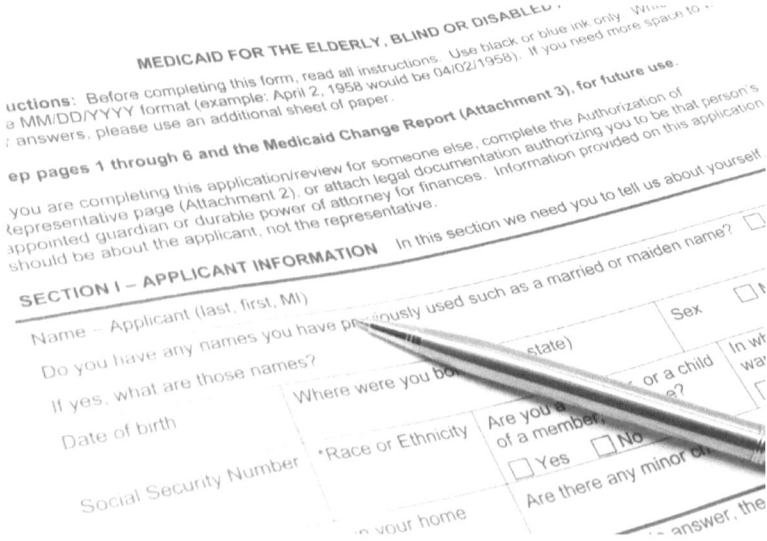

Then, go to the front desk and ask them for a Medicaid Application and any appropriate forms that need to be submitted with it. In some states, if someone else is applying on your behalf, you will need to complete a form appointing this person as your Authorized Representative. In those states that pose an income cap for the nursing home resident, they may have their own forms, which will need to be completed.

In most states, if you are looking for retroactive Medicaid eligibility coverage, you will need a separate application form that allows you to apply for up to three (3) months of back coverage.

Let's use the example of Mr. and Mrs. Smith: Mrs. Smith has been in a nursing home and she has been privately paying for the months of July, August and September. In the month of October, Mr. Smith is just getting around to applying for his wife.

Assuming they have met all of the eligibility criteria for those months—and assuming that they are located in a state that allows them to be eligible for benefits if all eligibility criteria is met ANYTIME within said month—they would be able to apply for retroactive eligibility as of July. This option for retroactive eligibility is a huge benefit, and one that is often overlooked when applying for Medicaid. Such costly mistakes can be avoided, which underscores the importance of consulting with a Medicaid Planning Specialist before applying for Medicaid.

The Post-Application Process

After the Medicaid application has been submitted—with all of the proper documentation and proofs attached, which usually include five years of bank statements, tax returns, copies of all property and automobile titles, copies of all medical insurance cards, copies of all personal information (i.e., birth certificate, social security card, marriage license, etc.), also copies of any owned trusts, copies or verification of all income, copies of medical, property and utility expenses, and more—the caseworker will then process the application, confirming and verifying that everything is in 'good order'. This may entail further work on your end by explaining, for example, the circumstances behind certain bank transactions. Or, you may be asked to supply additional verifications.

Please note that if you fail to comply with **any** of the caseworker's verification requests, the caseworker will issue a Notice of Denial, and you will need to start the process all over again. This can end up costing you possibly months worth of Medicaid coverage, depending on your timing.

Once a Medicaid application has been approved, and assuming there is a community spouse involved, there is a certain time limit (depending on the state) as to when all transfers of title to the community spouse must be made. These transfers include those involving the house, bank accounts, investment accounts, life insurance policies—all assets that were kept as part of the community spouse's resource allowance, or as part of his or her exempt assets—and all of these need to be completed on time.

As mentioned before, the nursing home resident is only allowed a small resource allowance of typically $2,000 in his or her name. If any asset over that amount is still held in his or her name, then Medicaid can retroactively deny eligibility for each and every month that person was considered over-resourced.

At the same time, Medicaid will conduct an annual review every year to re-determine your Medicaid eligibility. You will be required to submit verifications of assets and income for the prior year. The caseworker will need to determine that the Medicaid applicant remained under the resource limitation at all times. The caseworker will also need to determine that the applicant did not acquire any additional assets or income.

General Information Regarding Medicaid

Other things you should know about Medicaid include age requirements for qualification.

Generally, you must be 65, or you may be under 65 if disabled.

Children under 6 may be Medicaid-eligible if the family household income falls beneath $133% of the federally designated poverty level. Medicaid also covers under-21 prenatal care, and it provides certain levels of care including vaccines, pediatrics and family nursing, delivery, pediatric follow-up, periodic screenings/diagnostics and treatment for children under the age of 21—if they meet federal poverty-level requirements.

Basically, all medical bills, most prescription drugs, hospitals stays and nursing care are covered by Medicaid. Other services must include in-patient and outpatient hospital services, physician services, medical and surgical dental, nursing facility services, in-home care, lab and x-ray services and family nurse-practitioner services. (Medicare will pick up part of these costs within the first 100 days of care).

What MAY be covered according to options offered state by state: ambulatory services, meaning assistance getting around with scooters and wheel chairs, getting in and out of bed, etc. Additional options may apply to prescription drug coverage and/or include optometry services and eyeglasses, prosthetic devices, regular dental services and in-home assistance.

Regarding in-home, adult day-care and other services, it is always wise to keep a log of specific types of care that have been used, and their specific costs along with dates and even specific times when such care had been applied. Also, keep a log of prescription drugs and supplemental health care supplies (bandages, etc.) used over a period of time. These records may come in handy if the in-home patient has a change of health and requires more extensive care from Medicaid.

#

PARTING COMMENTS

I F YOU HAVE been reading my book under the sometimes monumental stress of placing someone in a nursing home on Medicaid, know that you are not alone. Millions of Americans have successfully navigated the process and by using some or all of the information included here, you now have a real heads-up, head-start in the Medicaid planning process.

Knowledge and understanding are the keys to opening doors with Medicaid people all over the country and they are not there to work against you. They are there to help you find your way to a solution best suited for you and your family as quickly possible, without incurring unnecessary expenses along the way.

After reading this book, you also know that you will need to step up and do more than just walk through the door of your local Medicaid office and expect solutions to magically appear. You will need to help them process your case in the most cordial and efficient manner possible, through the kind of advance preparation mentioned throughout the book.

Yet, now you know which documents to have prepared in advance. You know the way assets are counted and under what circumstances property and other matters will be considered under Medicaid guidelines. You also know that nothing is perfect in an imperfect world.

As I have said throughout the book, because no two caseworkers are alike and because no two personal situations will precisely align with one another, you may need guidance from time to time, especially when complex legal and/or financial matters are involved. *That's* the real secret to Medicaid planning: knowing when to bring in a pro for a bit of consultation and when to go it alone. A brief session with the right attorney, for example, may save countless, frustrating hours of dealing with the wrong people in the wrong places, all of whom are trying to help but who may lack the information you need.

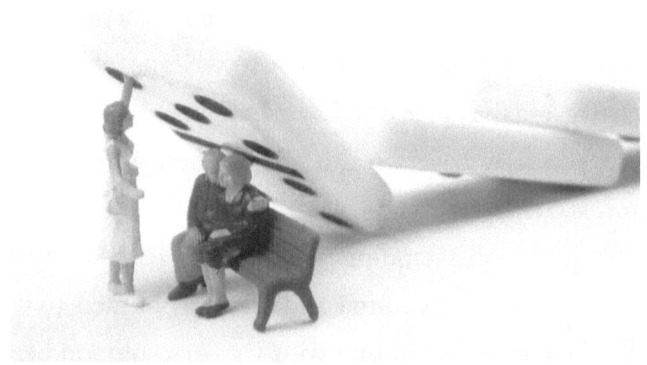

The basic rule of thumb when you reach a stumbling block is simple: *When you don't know, don't go* without some outside help. Most people don't even know that Medicaid specialists exist! Now you do, and all I can say from personal experience is that the relatively modest professional fees you may spend in the beginning may save you hundreds or even hundreds of thousands of dollars in the end.

As happens for a great many people armed with information provided here, your Medicaid planning process may be simple and streamlined, requiring no additional assistance whatsoever. Still, if you are entering the process for the first time, or if you anticipate doing so in the near future, I suggest having a team of specialists in place, should you run into seemingly impassable barriers along the way.

CHERYL L. FLETCHER-DOCHERTY

Whatever your situation may be, please feel free to contact me anytime if you have any questions or problems. My door is always open, solutions are available for almost any situation, which means that Medicaid nightmares can turn into dream solutions once you have the right stuff for the job.

All my best to you and your loved ones.
Sincerely,
Cheryl L. Fletcher-Docherty

www.ingramcontent.com/pod-product-compliance
Lightning Source LLC
Chambersburg PA
CBHW021235280526
45784CB00005B/2112